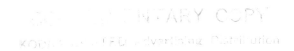
Contents

Introduction

X-rays

X-rays are produced when fast-moving electrons collide with matter. The following of their properties are of significance to the dental radiographer:
1) They can penetrate matter to an extent dependent on its density and thickness.
2) They travel in straight lines.
3) They can produce a developable image on film.
4) They can produce changes, both somatic and genetic, in living tissues.
5) When they impinge on matter, some of the rays are scattered in random directions.
6) They are not detectable by the human senses.

The first three of these properties are useful in radiography; the last three necessitate great caution in the use of X-rays.

Dental X-ray equipment

The dental X-ray tube (see Figure 1) is an evacuated glass envelope containing a cathode (the source of the electrons), and an anode (the target or focus at which they are directed). The electrons are emitted from a heated filament within the cathode, and are accelerated from the cathode to the anode by a very high voltage applied between the two. From the target area of the anode, X-rays are emitted in all directions.

The tube is surrounded by a heavy metal housing that absorbs all the X-rays except for a narrow beam, which is allowed to escape through a window or portal. The beam is further limited, to the minimum area necessary for the work being done, by a diaphragm. This is a heavy-metal disc with a circular hole, which can be fitted in front of the tube window. The window is also covered with an aluminium filter, which absorbs the least-penetrating X-rays; these would otherwise be absorbed or scattered by the patient's skin.

The plastics cone fitted in front of the tube is merely a positioning device and has no focusing or directional action on the X-ray beam. The point of the cone indicates the middle of the X-ray beam, normally termed the central ray.

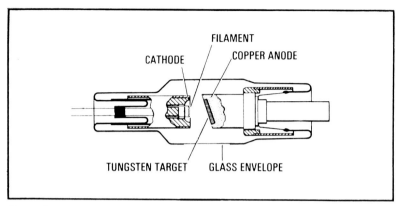

FILAMENT

CATHODE COPPER ANODE

TUNGSTEN TARGET GLASS ENVELOPE

Figure 1

The action of the electron beam striking the target gives rise to great heat; the tungsten target is therefore embedded in a copper block, which conducts the heat rapidly away to an oil jacket surrounding the tube. The heat is dissipated through the outer casing.

The high voltage necessary for the tube's operation is supplied by a transformer; in most dental X-ray machines the voltage is fixed at a value of 50 to 60kV (1kV=1000 volts). The tube current is normally also fixed, at a value between 7 and 10mA (1mA=0.001 amp).

Operation of dental X-ray machines

With the majority of dental X-ray machines, the exposure is controlled solely by a mechanical or electronic timer that will switch on the X-ray beam for a pre-selected length of time. The other factors that can affect exposure are all fixed: the high voltage (kilovoltage) and the current (milliamperage) are standard for the machine, and, for most intra-oral work, the distance from the tube focus to the X-ray film is kept constant by making all exposures with the cone almost in contact with the patient's skin. This last point is an important one, since exposure varies as the square of the focus-to-film distance, and therefore a small change in the focus-to-film distance has a considerable effect on the exposure. It also follows that the exposure time chosen will depend on the type of machine being used, since electrical settings and cone length vary from one type to another. Further guidance on this will be found under the heading "Exposure factors" on page 5.

Once the correct exposure time has been determined, the operating sequence is straightforward:
a) The filament-heating current is switched on.
b) The exposure time is set.
c) The film is positioned.

d) The patient's head is positioned.
e) The tube is positioned.
f) The automatic timer is operated to make the exposure.

The hazards associated with X-rays make it essential to adhere to a set safety procedure. This will be dealt with next.

Safety procedure

The following precautions are aimed at reducing to a minimum the X-ray exposure to patient and operator.

To reduce exposure to the patient:

1) The X-ray film employed should be a "fast" type, such as KODAK Fast Dental X-ray Film.
2) The X-ray tube should be fitted with a diaphragm which limits the width of the beam to the minimum necessary to cover the area under examination. It should not exceed 6cm in diameter at the tip of the cone and MUST not exceed 7.5cm in diameter.
3) The X-ray tube should be so fitted that total filtration must be equivalent to not less than 1.5mm aluminium for voltages up to and including 70kV.
4) The number of exposures made should be the minimum necessary for diagnosis. A competent operator should avoid the necessity for repeat exposures.
5) If views are taken that could involve the direct irradiation of the gonads or a foetus then the patient should wear a protective apron equivalent to 0.25mm of lead.
6) Correct film processing is essential to produce good quality radiographs and to avoid repeat films.

To reduce exposure to the operator and staff:

1) The operator must not stand in the direct beam during exposure.
2) The operator must stand at least one metre from the tube and patient during exposure when using equipment of up to 70kV.
3) The tube housing, cone or the film must not be held by the operator or other staff during exposure.
4) Routine checks on the performance and safety requirements of X-ray equipment should be carried out.

Advice on radiation checks can be obtained from the National Radiological Protection Board who operate a postal scheme for checking equipment.

For further advice consult: *Radiological Protection in Dental Practice*, prepared by the Standing Dental Advisory Committee and issued by the Department of Health and Social Security, March 1975.

Intra-oral radiography

General considerations

The following points apply to all three types of intra-oral radiographic examination – periapical, interproximal and occlusal:

Films

Kodak Limited offers the following types of film for intra-oral radiography.

For use without a cassette:

KODAK Fast Dental X-ray Film

reference number	*size*	*packing*
Periapical		
4S–50	$1\frac{1}{4} \times 1\frac{5}{8}$ in (3.2×4.1 cm)	50 singles
4S–150	$1\frac{1}{4} \times 1\frac{5}{8}$ in (3.2×4.1 cm)	150 singles
5P–50	$1\frac{1}{4} \times 1\frac{5}{8}$ in (3.2×4.1 cm)	50 pairs
5P–150	$1\frac{1}{4} \times 1\frac{5}{8}$ in (3.2×4.1 cm)	150 pairs
'Bite-Wing' Films		
BW–2	$1\frac{1}{4} \times 1\frac{5}{8}$ in (3.2×4.1 cm)	25 singles
In KODAK 'Dentech' Pack		
Periapical		
D0–50	22×35 mm	50 singles
D4–100	31×41 mm	100 singles
Occlusal		
D3–25	57×76 mm	25 singles

KODAK Ultra-Speed Dental X-ray Film

Occlusal		
DF–46	$2\frac{1}{4} \times 3$ in (5.7×7.6 cm)	10 singles
Periapical		
DF–51	$\frac{7}{8} \times 1\frac{3}{8}$ in (2.2×3.5 cm)	50 singles
'Bite-Wing'		
DF–42	$1\frac{1}{16} \times 2\frac{1}{8}$ in (2.7×5.4 cm)	25 singles

KODAK 'Defilux' Dental X-ray Film

For subdued white light processing

	3.1×4.1 cm	150 singles

For use with an intra-oral cassette and intensifying screens:

KODAK 'RP X-Omat' Medical X-ray Film

size	*sheets per box*	*packing*
$2\frac{1}{4} \times 3$ in $(5.7 \times 7.6$ cm$)$	50	interleaved

Preliminary inspection

A preliminary examination should be made of the patient's mouth and dentition, since variations in the shape of the dental arches and irregularities in tooth growth may necessitate important deviations from the standard radiographic technique. In the partially edentulous jaw, careful identification of the remaining teeth is important in order that the correct tube angulation and exposure are selected. If the patient is wearing spectacles, they should be removed, as should dentures unless they assist in retention of the film packet.

Positioning the film packet

Proper positioning of the film packet is necessary in order to avoid excessive bending, which leads to distortion of the image (Figure 2), and movement of the packet during exposure, which causes blurring (Figure 3). The adoption of a standard packet position for each region will ensure that serial radiographs are comparable with one another.

All KODAK intra-oral X-ray films are supplied in packets with a pebbled anti-slip surface on one side, which is known as the tube side. The anti-slip surface is placed next to the region to be exposed. Each film has an embossed dot, raised on the tube side, to assist in orienting the radiograph when it is being mounted.

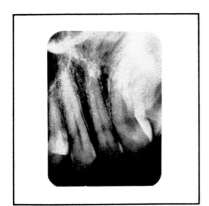

Figure 2

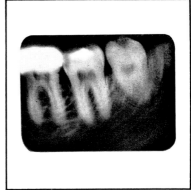

Figure 3

In placing the packet in the patient's mouth:
1) Avoid sliding the packet into position. Irritation of the oral mucosa often causes retching.
2) Hold the packet in position until the patient is holding it securely. *The dentist or his assistant should never hold the packet in position during an exposure.*

Some patients have a tendency to retch when a film packet is placed in the mouth. A careful explanation of the procedure will help a nervous patient to relax and to overcome this tendency. Deep breathing through the mouth also helps to minimize retching, especially during the examination of the molar areas.

Positioning the patient's head

In positioning the patient for the radiographic exposure, attention should be paid to the adjustment of the chair-back and neck-rest so that the patient can maintain the correct position with comfort. This is important in reducing the possibility of movement by the patient during the exposure.

Angulation of the X-ray tube

The vertical angle set on the scale of the X-ray tube is the angle between the central ray of the X-ray beam and the horizontal. It is given as a positive figure when the central ray intersects the horizontal from above and a negative figure when the intersection is from below.

Immobilization

Movement of the patient or the X-ray tube during exposure has an adverse effect on image sharpness. The operator should make sure that the tube is stationary before the exposure is made and should also observe the patient. If the patient's breathing causes the head to move, the exposure should be made while he is holding his breath.

Exposure factors

The exposure times given in this book are applicable to the examination of the average adult patient, using a dental X-ray machine of output 60kV and 10mA and, except where otherwise stated, a focus-to-film distance of 9 inches (23cm). For the examination of children the exposure is reduced by approximately 30 per cent, and for edentulous patients by approximately 40 per cent.

If the machine used has an output other than 60kV/10mA, the exposure time must be adjusted accordingly.

The periapical examination

Purpose

To examine the formation and condition of the entire tooth and its surrounding alveolar tissues. It is particularly useful for studying the apices of the teeth.

The complete periapical radiographic examination provides the dentist with a comprehensive record that is a diagnostic aid and a basis for the planning of treatment. Individual dental radiographs reveal conditions requiring treatment and are a reliable aid to the choice of procedure.

For the patient who has not previously had a dental X-ray examination, it may be advisable to begin with a complete periapical study, starting with the maxillary central-incisor region and then proceeding to the remaining maxillary regions. After the upper incisor regions have been examined, the patient will have become accustomed to the procedure and should co-operate more readily during the more difficult examination of the molar regions. Accordingly, our detailed description of the periapical examination deals first with the anterior and then with the posterior regions. The standard procedure for each region gives detailed instructions for the positioning of the film packet.

Film requirements

The central regions of the maxilla and the mandible can each be recorded in one film. A minimum of 5 or 6 radiographs is needed in each arch: 2 central-lateral incisor, 2 canine-premolar, 2 molar. Thus, the basic full-mouth examination for the average adult patient consists of 11 radiographs – 6 maxillary and 5 mandibular. Because of anatomical interference in the anterior maxillary area, an additional view of each canine region may be desirable for some patients. On the other hand, the complete examination can at times be accomplished with only ten films.

Some patients have such narrow dental arches that the full size packets cannot be placed in the anterior areas without excessive bending. In such situations, the smaller "0" size packets can be used. The dental radiographic examination of a child requires a smaller film packet, in order that the patient should be comfortable and the film flat. In this case, one "0" size packet is used for each central-lateral incisor, canine and molar region.

Positioning the periapical film packet

The best radiographs are obtained when the film is kept as flat as possible. It will help in this respect if the patient is asked to support the packet by placing a finger behind the film pressing gently on to the crown of the tooth. It is permissible to bend the corner of the packet as an aid to correct positioning and the patient's comfort.

Head positions

For periapical examinations of both the upper and lower jaws, the head should be supported with the median plane vertical. For a periapical examination of either jaw, **the occlusal plane of that jaw should be horizontal.** As visualization of the angle of the occlusal plane is difficult, a base line can be taken between two superficial anatomical landmarks known to be parallel to the occlusal plane.

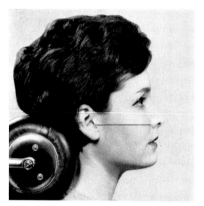
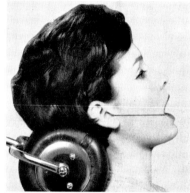

Figure 4   Figure 5

Normally, the maxillary occlusal plane is horizontal when a line drawn from the tragus of the ear to the ala of the nose is horizontal (Figure 4), and the mandibular occlusal plane is horizontal when the mouth is open and a line drawn from the tragus of the ear to the corner of the mouth is horizontal (Figure 5 shows the head position). However, if the preliminary examination reveals an abnormal relationship between the occlusal plane and these external landmarks, allowance for this should be made in positioning.

Central-ray projection: vertical angle

To produce an accurate image of a tooth in a periapical radiograph, the central ray must be projected perpendicularly to a plane bisecting the angle formed by the longitudinal axis of the tooth and the plane of the film packet. By following this principle, an average vertical angle can be estimated for each area. The head of the X-ray machine carries a scale of vertical angles for ready reference. Figure 6 shows correct angulation, together with the resulting radiograph. Figures 7 and 8 show incorrect angulation and the resulting elongated and foreshortened images.

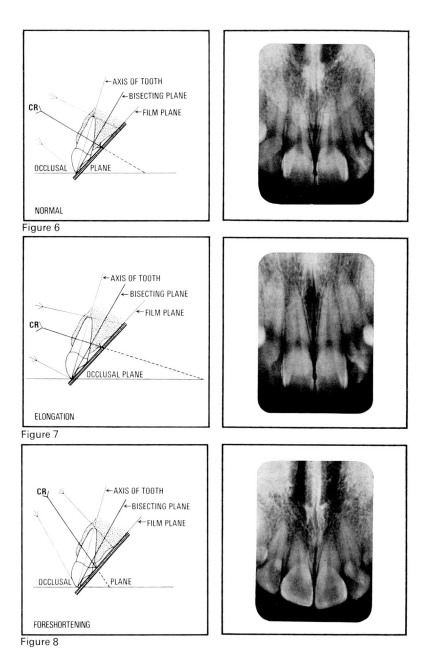

Figure 6

Figure 7

Figure 8

Average vertical angles can be used in the majority of cases, because most jaws are reasonably symmetrical. Figure 9 shows the normal vertical angle of $+20°$ for an average vault. When, in the maxillary region, a high vault causes the film packet to assume a more vertical

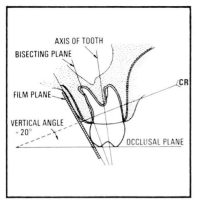

Figure 9

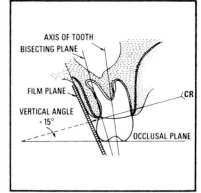

Figure 10

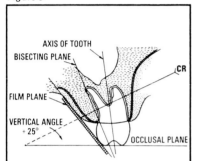

Figure 11

position, the vertical angle is *decreased* by 5° (Figure 10). For a low vault, the vertical angle is *increased* by 5° (Figure 11).

In the mandibular region, the vertical angle is *increased* by 5° from the normal when the teeth are buccally inclined or the floor of the mouth is shallower than average; it is *decreased* by 5° when the teeth are more vertical or the mouth deeper than average.

Central-ray projection: horizontal angle

The central ray must be projected through the interproximal spaces in order that the images of the teeth shall not overlap one another. This is illustrated in Figures 12 and 13, which show correct and incorrect horizontal angles and the resulting radiographs.

Figure 14 shows the recommended average vertical and horizontal angles for the complete periapical examination.

Supplementary views are often necessary, as in the localization of impacted teeth, when the standard projection angles may be varied to produce additional specific information.

12

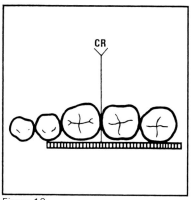
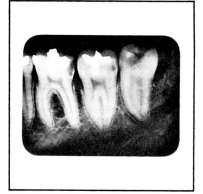

Figure 12

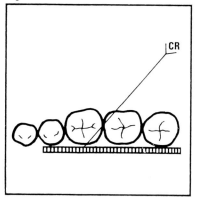
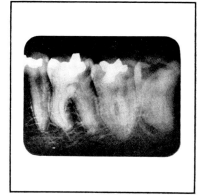

Figure 13

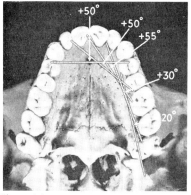
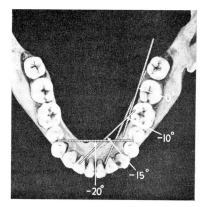

Figure 14

Exposure factors (examples)

Tube factors – tube rating – average rating 10mA 60kV
  – anode/film distance – inverse square law applies
  – voltage fluctuations – variations in input should be compensated

Film factors – fast film/slow film – exposure varies according to film sensitivity
  – non screen film/screen film – intra-oral film is normally non-screen, screen film used in cassettes fitted with intensifying screens

Patient factors – calibrate normal range of exposures for normal adult with full teeth.

Adjustments in exposure should be made as follows:

– periodontal examination – 3/4 normal
– children under 8–10 yrs – 2/3 normal
– edentulous patients – 1/2 normal
– Pathology – cysts etc. – 1/2 normal
  – osteoma etc. – 2x normal

Maxillary incisor region

Approximate exposure: 0.25 second.

Packet position: long axis in a vertical plane, lower edge about $\frac{1}{8}$ inch below edges of teeth.

Average vertical angle: +50°.

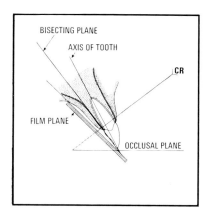

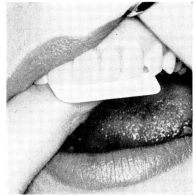

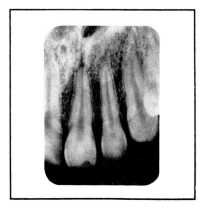

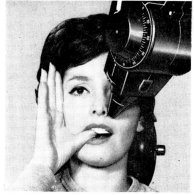

Maxillary pre-molar region

Approximate exposure: 0.35 second.

Packet position: long axis horizontal, lower edge about $\frac{1}{8}$ inch below edges of teeth.

Average vertical angle: $+30°$.

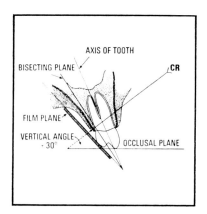

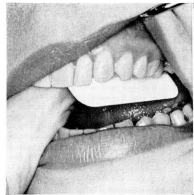

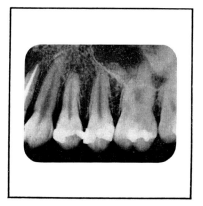

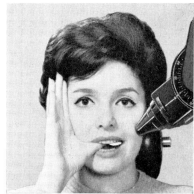

Maxillary molar region

Approximate exposure: 0.5 second.

Packet position: long axis horizontal, anterior edge distal of first pre-molar, lower edge about $\frac{1}{8}$ inch below edges of teeth.

Average vertical angle: $+20°$.

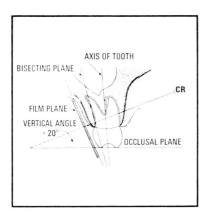

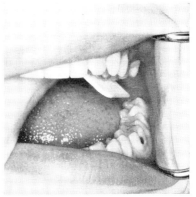

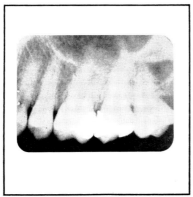

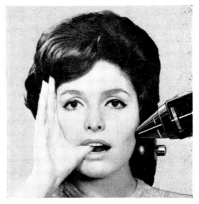

Mandibular incisor region

Approximate exposure: 0.25 second.

Packet position: long axis horizontal, upper edge about $\frac{1}{8}$ inch above edges of teeth.

Average vertical angle: $-20°$.

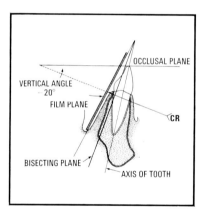

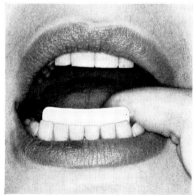

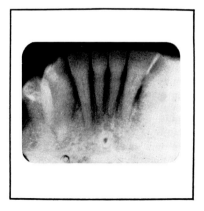

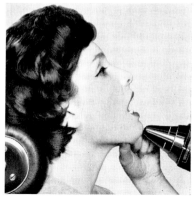

Mandibular pre-molar region

Approximate exposure: 0.25 second.

Packet position: long axis horizontal, upper edge about $\frac{1}{8}$ inch above edges of teeth.

Average vertical angle: $-10°$.

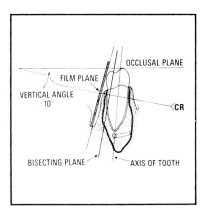

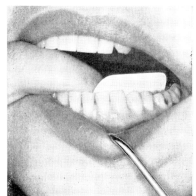

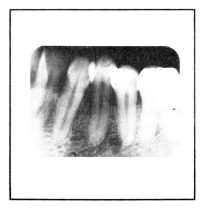

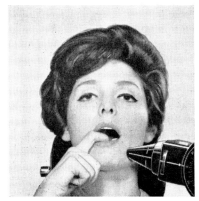

Mandibular molar region

Approximate exposure: 0.35 second.

Packet position: long axis horizontal, upper edge about $\frac{1}{8}$ inch above edges of teeth.

Average vertical angle: $-0°$.

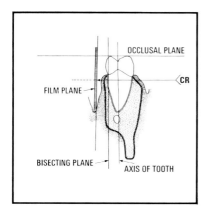

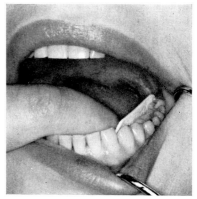

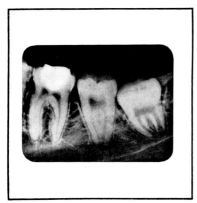

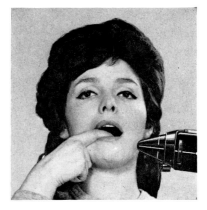

The interproximal examination

Purpose

Caries on the exposed surfaces of the teeth can be detected by the usual visual and instrumental methods, but caries concealed on the interproximal surfaces is more difficult to detect, particularly when it affects posterior teeth of large buccolingual diameter. The interproximal radiographic examination with 'Bite-Wing' Film can often be useful in such cases.

This method of examination reveals interproximal and occlusal caries, pulp size and pulp changes, overhanging restorations, recurrent caries under existing restorations, improperly fitted artificial crowns and the height of the alveolar crest.

Figure 15
'Bite-wing'
Film packet

It has an advantage over the periapical examination in that images of the coronal and cervical portions of both the upper and lower teeth, and the alveolar borders of a given region, can all be recorded on a single film.

Head position

The patient's head is positioned so that the occlusal plane of the maxillary teeth is horizontal at the time of the exposure (see Figure 4, page 10).

Positioning the 'Bite-Wing' Film packet

In standardized interproximal techniques the packet is placed in a definite position for each region, so that the plane of the film is nearly parallel to the interdental axes of the crowns of the teeth; the tab, or wing, is retained between the occluded teeth. The correct position of the packet is maintained by holding the wing while the patient gently bites on to it.

Central-ray projection

In the interproximal examination, the central ray is projected approximately perpendicular to the film and through the points of contact of the teeth. A low maxillary vault may cause the packet to assume a less upright position; a slight downward angulation of the central ray will then be necessary to make it perpendicular to the film.

Pre-molar—molar region

Approximate exposure: 0.3 second.

Packet position: centre level with first molar teeth.

Average vertical angle: −0°.

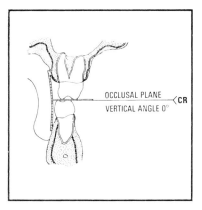

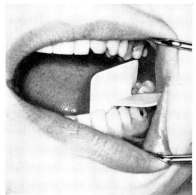

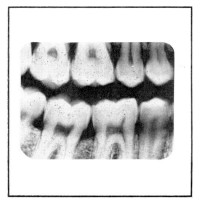

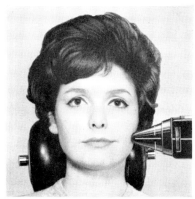

The occlusal examination

Purpose

Occlusal radiography – so called because the film packet is placed in the occlusal plane for exposure – is a supplementary procedure for showing large dental areas on a single film. The occlusal radiograph reveals conditions that often cannot be recorded conveniently on any other film.

The uses of occlusal radiography include the rapid surveying of teeth and jaws for locating impacted teeth, foreign bodies and calculi in the salivary ducts; locating and determining the extent of such lesions as cysts, osteomyelitis and malignancies; recording changes in the size and shape of the dental arches; detecting supernumerary teeth; observing the condition of the upper jaw following operations for the closure of a cleft palate; and examining edentulous areas, which frequently are the site of local infection from root fragments, cystic growths, necrotic areas, etc. In cases of trauma, if the patient's mouth can be opened enough for the insertion of the packet, the occlusal radiograph is very useful in demonstrating fractures of the palatine and alveolar processes of the maxilla and various parts of the mandible.

The intra-oral cassette

Occlusal radiography for the location of unerupted maxillary teeth can be facilitated by the use of an intra-oral cassette equipped with X-ray intensifying screens (Figure 16). The shorter exposure times permitted by the screen technique minimize the possibility of movement of the subject during exposure and consequent blur of the radiographic image.

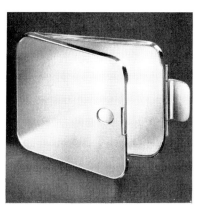

Figure 16

Head positions

For the maxillary occlusal examination, the head is positioned so that the line from the tragus of the ear to the ala of the nose is horizontal (see Figure 4, page 10).

The head positions for the occlusal examination of the mandibular areas vary with the region being examined.

Positioning the occlusal film packet or cassette

The packet is positioned in the mouth with its short axis coincident with the median plane. The occlusal cassette, due to its bulk, may be positioned with its long axis coincident with the median plane, and will require to be marked "L" or "R" prior to exposure.

The patient closes the mouth and immobilizes the film packet with a gentle edge to edge bite.

The cassette should be supported manually by the patient, who should be instructed not to bite on it.

Central-ray projection

The direction of the central ray is dependent on the region being examined; specific details are given individually for each type of occlusal examination.

Maxillary region – (Standard occlusal view)

Approximate exposure: 0.3 second.

Packet position: short axis coincident with median plane.

Central-ray direction: through bridge of nose; average vertical angle +65°.

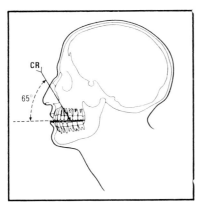

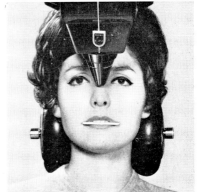

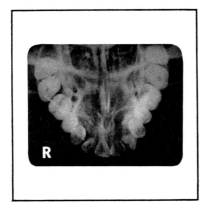

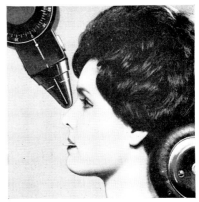

Maxillary canine—molar region – (Oblique occlusal view)

Approximate exposure: 0.3 second.

Packet position: short axis coincident with median plane; posterior edge against ramus of mandible.

Central-ray direction: through canine fossa; vertical angle +60°, horizontal angle 60° to median plane.

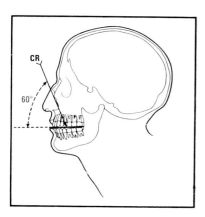

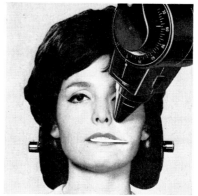

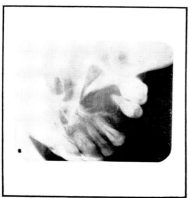

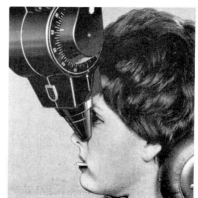

Location of maxillary teeth – vertex occlusal projection (with cassette)

Approximate exposure: 1.0 second.

Focus-to-film distance: 16 inches.

Cassette position: long axis in median plane; posterior edge against rami of mandible.

Central-ray direction: through coronal suture, towards centre of cassette. Vertical angle +75° (forwards).

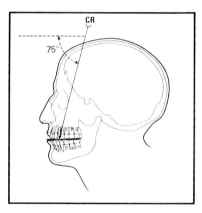
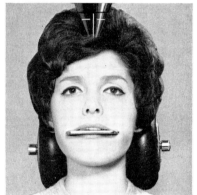
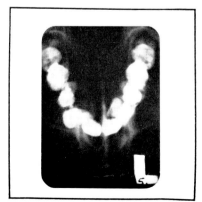
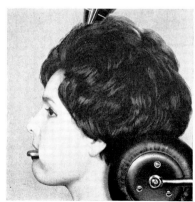

Entire lower arch – (Standard occlusal view)

Approximate exposure: 0.5 second.

Packet position: short axis in median plane; posterior edge against rami of mandible.

Head position: occlusal plane of maxillary teeth vertical.

Central-ray direction: towards centre of packet. Vertical angle 90°.

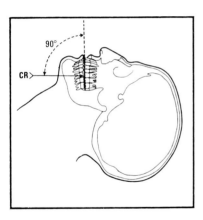
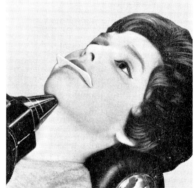
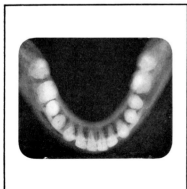
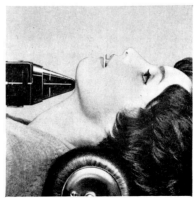

Mandibular molar region – (Oblique occlusal view)

Approximate exposure: 0.5 second.

Packet position: short axis in median plane; posterior edge against ramus of mandible.

Head position: occlusal plane vertical.

Central-ray direction: towards centre of packet. Vertical angle 90°.

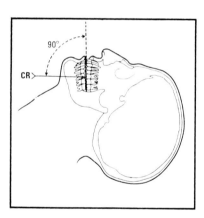

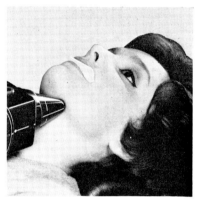

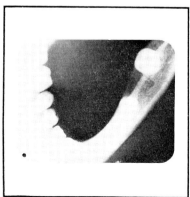

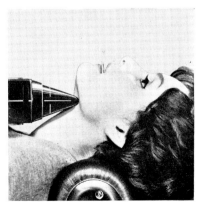

Extra-oral radiography

General considerations

Extra-oral radiography, whilst not a substitute for the intra-oral X-ray examination, supplements the information obtained from periapical, interproximal and occlusal radiographs. It is especially valuable in the examination of the mandible, the maxilla, the temporo-mandibular joints and the facial profile. There are many projections in common use; we have recorded only one for each region.

Films

For extra-oral work, KODAK 'RP X-Omat' Medical X-ray Film, exposed between Intensifying Screens, offers satisfactory speed, wide exposure latitude and dependable uniformity: properties that are of great importance in recording fine detail with good contrast. The exposure times recommended in the following section apply to this film.

Non-screen films, such as KODIREX X-ray Film, may need **ten times as much exposure as screen-type films;** they are not, therefore, recommended where it is vital to minimize the X-ray dose to the patient. An isolated exception to this is in facial-profile radiography, where KODIREX X-ray Film can be used to demonstrate the soft-tissue outline: in this case, both screen-type and non-screen films receive the same exposure.

All sizes of KODAK 'RP X-Omat' Medical X-ray Film are supplied in interleaved packs. The following sizes are most commonly used in dental radiography.

KODAK 'RP X-Omat' Medical X-ray Film.

Size (inches)	sheets per box
$2\frac{1}{4} \times 3$ (occlusal)	50
$4\frac{3}{4} \times 6\frac{1}{2}$	100
(centimetres)	
13×18	100

Larger sizes are available.

Preparation of film for exposure

Screen-type X-ray films for extra-oral radiography are not wrapped in light-tight packets as are intra-oral films. Instead, they are packed in boxes, each sheet of film in a folder of protective interleaving paper. The boxes are designed to provide easy film removal. It is very important that X-ray film is handled *only* under safelighting conditions. For X-ray films, a KODAK Safelamp fitted with a 25W pearl lamp and the correct filter must be used. KODAK Safelight Filter No.6B or GS-1 (minimum distance from film, 4 feet) and KODAK Safelight Filter No.OA (minimum distance from film via reflecting surface, 7 feet) are suitable.

After the box has been opened and the required films loaded into the exposure holders or cassettes, the lid of the box must be replaced before the white light is switched on.

Loading exposure holder or cassette

X-ray sheet film must be handled carefully to avoid damage due to pressure, creasing, buckling and friction. Cassettes should be loaded only in the darkroom after the white light has been switched off and the safelamp turned on. Interleaving paper *must be removed* before the film is placed in the cassette (Figure 17). For exposure holders, however, the film should be left in the interleaving paper.

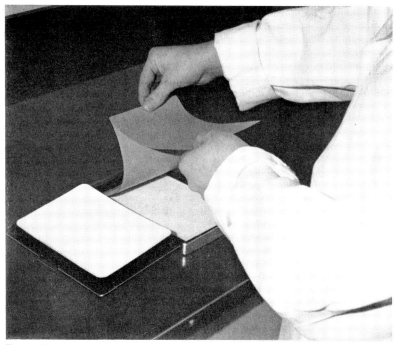

Figure 17

Oblique jaw view – for molar region

Approximate exposure: 0.25 second.

Intensifying screens: medium speed.

Focus-to-film distance: 15 inches.

Patient position: sitting sideways, arm of dental chair being lowered.

Cassette position: resting on head-rest and chair-back, film at 45° to horizontal. Patient holds cassette at lower corners.

Head position: zygomatic arch touching cassette, lower border of mandible parallel to its bottom edge.

Central-ray direction: centre from a point one inch behind angle of mandible, towards opposite mid-molar region. Vertical angle perpendicular to cassette.

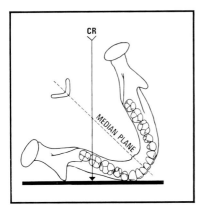
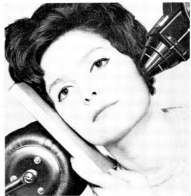

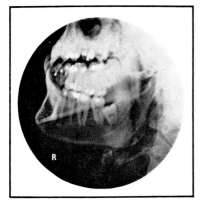

Oblique jaw view – for premolar region

Approximate exposure: 0.25 second.

Intensifying screens: medium speed.

Focus-to-film distance: 15 inches.

Patient position: sitting sideways, arm of dental chair being lowered.

Cassette position: resting on head-rest and chair-back, film at 45° to horizontal. Patient holds cassette at lower corners.

Head position: canine/premolar region touching centre of cassette, lower border of mandible parallel to its bottom edge.

Central-ray direction: centre from a point one inch behind angle of mandible through canine/premolar teeth. Vertical angle perpendicular to cassette.

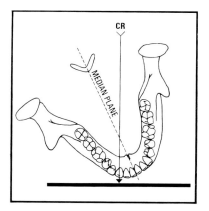
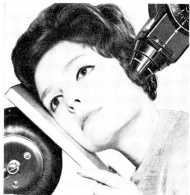

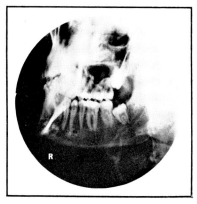

True lateral face view

Approximate exposure: 0.5 second.

Intensifying screens: medium speed.

Focus-to-film distance: approx. 16 inches.

Cassette position: vertical, parallel to median plane.

Head position: median plane vertical.

Central-ray direction: horizontal through canine region.

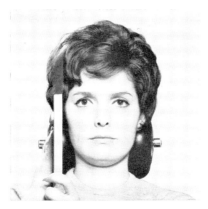

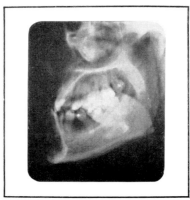

Extra-oral views not normally taken on a dental unit.

Mandible (postero-anterior)

Approximate exposure: 50mAs.

Intensifying screens: medium speed.

Focus-to-film distance: 30 inches.

Cassette position: horizontal or vertical, according to equipment used.

Head position: nose and forehead touching cassette. Median plane vertical.

Central-ray direction: through point $2\frac{1}{2}$ inches below external occipital protuberance, in mid-line, at 90° to film.

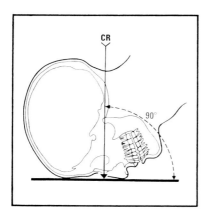

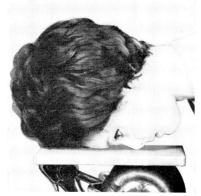

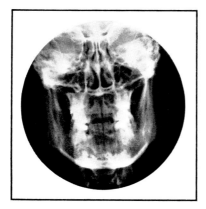

NOTE: Facial Maxillary examinations are best carried out using equipment of higher power than that for intra-oral examinations. This enables the use of shorter exposures, thus limiting unsharpness due to movement of the patient.

Temporo-mandibular articulation

Approximate exposure: 50mAs.

Intensifying screens: medium speed.

Focus-to-film distance: 30 inches.

Patient position: median plane horizontal or vertical according to equipment used.

Cassette position: horizontal or vertical as above.

Head position: true lateral.

Central-ray direction: through point one inch above and one inch behind external auditory meatus on tube side towards opposite temporo-mandibular joint. Vertical angle about +25°.

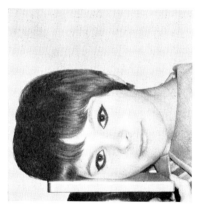
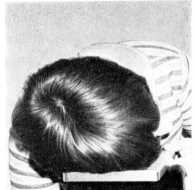

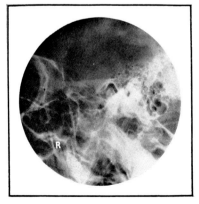

Panoramic radiography

The advantages of panoramic techniques in dental radiography are being developed for routine full mouth examinations.

The main advantage is that a record of a patient's complete dentition may be produced in a few seconds on one sheet of film; if any pathology requires more detailed examination, intra-oral or other views may be used in the normal way.

Kodak Limited provide RP/L X-OMAT Medical X-ray Film in two sizes, 12 cm × 30 cm and 15 cm × 30 cm.

The film must be handled and processed in a darkroom using a safelamp fitted with a 6B or GS-1 Filter.

The film may be processed in an automatic processor, or in tanks; these should be deep enough to accommodate the film in a suitable hanger. The process of development, fixing and washing are similar to those involved when using intra-oral films.

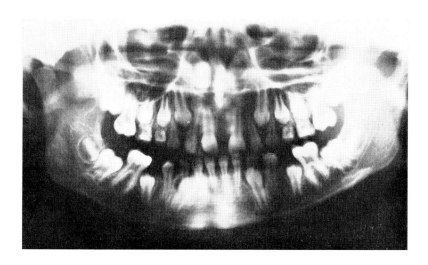

Processing

Correct exposure of the film is only part of the production of a good dental radiograph; processing the film completes the sequence, since it produces a lasting visible image from the latent image created by X-rays. Correct processing makes an essential contribution to the quality of the radiograph. The fundamental requirements for good processing are adequate equipment and a standardized procedure.

The darkroom

Standardization of processing procedure is so important that a separate darkroom should be a part of every dental suite. The principal requirements for an efficient darkroom are:
1) Absolute exclusion of external light.
2) Separate areas for wet and dry working.
3) Hot and cold water supplies.
4) Adequate space for the separate storage of film, chemicals and accessories.
5) Safelight and white-light illumination.

The darkroom should be as close as possible to the room where the radiographic examinations are performed, and for economy and easy installation its location should preferably take advantage of existing drainage, water and electrical supplies.

A room with floor space of about 8×6 feet will be satisfactory. The door must be light-tight and fitted with a catch to prevent intrusions while films are being handled.

The walls should preferably be painted a light colour with a high-gloss finish for brightness and cleanness. A white emulsion paint is recommended for the ceiling, and the floor should be covered with pvc tiles or sheeting.

The bench working surface should be thick linoleum and dark in colour, so that films are easily seen against it. The working area must be divided into two parts, a "dry" bench for handling dry films and a "wet" bench, incorporating a sink with hot and cold water supplies, for processing. The sink will be required to accommodate an assembly of processing tanks, around which water can be circulated as an aid to maintaining a constant working temperature of 20°C (68°F). There

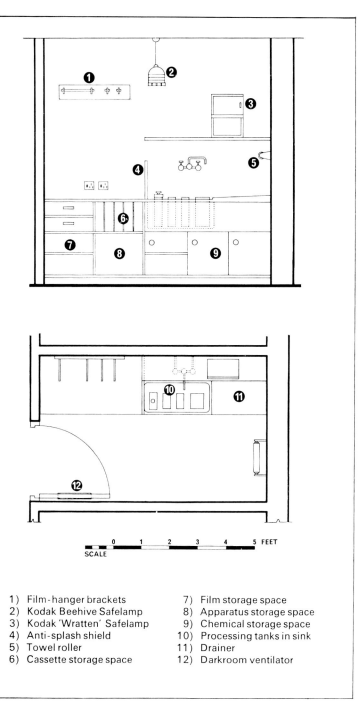

1) Film-hanger brackets
2) Kodak Beehive Safelamp
3) Kodak 'Wratten' Safelamp
4) Anti-splash shield
5) Towel roller
6) Cassette storage space

7) Film storage space
8) Apparatus storage space
9) Chemical storage space
10) Processing tanks in sink
11) Drainer
12) Darkroom ventilator

Figure 18. Plan of a typical dental X-ray darkroom

should be sufficient clearance between taps and sink to accommodate a bucket.

If space allows it, the wet and dry benches should be completely separate – for example, against opposite walls. Failing this, they must be separated by an effective anti-splash shield.

The dry bench should be approximately 3 feet high and 2 feet deep, and should incorporate a storage cupboard allowing chemicals and films to be stored completely separately from each other.

Equipment

Safelamps

An X-ray film will be fogged by excessive exposure to light, even if from a safelamp of a recommended type; therefore, care should be taken in the placing of safelamps in the darkroom. KODAK Safelamps are available as follows:

KODAK Beehive Safelamp (Figure 19)

For attachment to work-bench, shelf or wall, or suspension from ceiling.

KODAK 'Wratten' Safelamp (Figure 20)

For wall-mounting. Also functions as an illuminator for viewing radiographs.

KODAK Universal Safelamp Model 2 (Figure 21)

A hanging lamp for direct or indirect illumination.

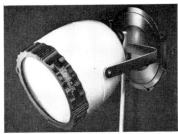

Figure 19

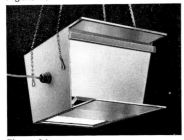

Figure 21

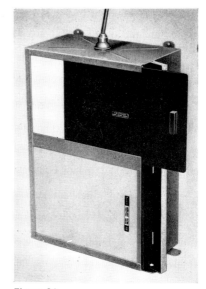

Figure 20

The recommended working conditions for various combinations of films and safelamps are given in the table below.

KODAK Safelamp	Beehive 'Wratten' or Universal	Universal
Type of illumination	Direct	Indirect
Rating of light bulb	25W	25W
Minimum safe working distance	4 feet	7 feet via reflecting surface
KODAK Safelight Filter Number recommended for: KODAK Fast Dental X-ray Film, and KODAK Ultra-Speed Dental X-ray Film	0A	0A
KODAK 'RP X-Omat' and 'RP/L X-Omat' Medical X-ray Film	6B or GS-1	0C
KODIREX X-ray Film	6B or GS-1	0C

NOTE: Safelamp illumination is not necessary for KODAK 'Defilux' Dental Film. The packet can be unwrapped in tungsten room lighting or subdued daylight.

If there is any doubt about the safety of the safelighting in the processing room, it can be tested easily. Open a dental film packet under safelamp illumination and place the film on the loading bench directly beneath the safelamp. Lay a small coin on the film. Leave the film exposed for one minute and process it in the usual way. If the outline of the coin is visible on the film, check the distance from lamp to bench and the wattage of the bulb. Also inspect the safelamp for damage and examine the filter for signs of deterioration.

Processing tanks

The tank method is a simple, effective way of processing X-ray films.

A complete set of tanks consists of three tanks for the developer, rinse and fixer and a larger tank for washing. The developer tank should be provided with a lid.

If 16 fl oz (455 ml) containers of KODAK Dental X-ray Developer or Fixer are used, a solution of the correct strength is obtained by emptying the container into an 80 fl oz (2.3 litres) tank and filling the tank almost to the top with water at the desired processing temperature.

In larger tank systems, the temperature of the solutions is thermo-statically controlled. There are also automatic systems, both large and small, for dental X-ray film processing.

Processing hangers

A range of film hangers in assorted sizes is indispensable in the dark-room. KODAK Dental Film Developing Hangers are available in two sizes for intra-oral films, holding ten or fourteen films properly spaced for tank processing. The hangers are of stainless steel and have white Ivorine identification tabs.

X-ray Processing Hangers are available in various sizes for sheet film. They are commonly of stainless steel with channelled sides and bottom, into which the film slides. The hinged top bar holds the film securely in place.

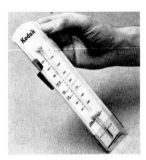

Figure 22

Thermometer

A thermometer is required. The KODAK Thermometer (Figure 22) is marked with both Celsius and Fahrenheit scales and has a detachable steel clip so that the thermometer can be hung in the tank.

Tank immersion heater

An immersion heater is needed to maintain a developer temperature of 20°C (68°F).

Timer

An alarm timer adjustable from 1 to 10 minutes should be available.

Illuminator

An illuminator for viewing wet radiographs is desirable in the dark-room. This saves carrying wet radiographs out of the processing room for examination.

Processing chemicals
Developer
This acts upon the invisible latent image produced in the film by X-rays or light from intensifying screens, and converts it into a visible image composed of minute particles of silver.

The following KODAK Developers are recommended for processing dental X-ray films:

KODAK Dental X-ray Developer – a concentrated liquid developer.

KODAK D-19 Developer Powder – suitable for all KODAK X-ray Films.

KODAK DX-80 Developer – a concentrated liquid developer especially recommended for tank processing.

KODAK Rapid Dental X-ray Developer – a liquid developer that is particularly recommended where a short processing time is desired: the development time is 30 seconds.

Developer replenisher
This is used, in the larger manual processing tanks, to compensate for the gradual decrease in chemical activity that occurs during processing. KODAK D-19R Replenisher Powder is made for replenishing solutions of D-19 Developer Powder, and KODAK DX-80R Replenisher may be added to solutions of DX-80 Developer.

Fixer
After development, the film must be cleared of undeveloped silver compounds that would otherwise darken under the action of light. This function is performed by the fixer, which also contains an ingredient that hardens the gelatin in the film so that it resists abrasion and can be dried by warm air without undue softening.

The following KODAK Fixing Chemicals are recommended for dental X-ray films:

KODAK Dental X-ray Fixer – a concentrated solution.

KODAK 'Unifix' Powder.

KODAK FX-40 X-ray Liquid Fixer.

Processing preliminaries
Processing the film makes the invisible latent image created by the X-rays visible and permanent. Good processing procedure, followed exactly, yields radiographs of uniform high quality. The steps in processing are development, rinse, fixing, washing and drying.

These steps will be dealt with in more detail in the following pages, but first there are some preliminary considerations.

Cleanliness

The liability of X-ray films to contamination makes cleanliness of prime importance in processing. It is imperative that the darkroom and equipment should be kept scrupulously clean and used only for their intended purpose.

Any spilt chemicals should be wiped up immediately so that they have no chance to dry, otherwise they may be carried into the air and deposited on film, causing spots. The thermometer and developing hangers should be washed thoroughly in clean water immediately after use, so that solutions adhering to them will not dry and later cause contaminated or streaked radiographs.

Preparation of solutions

The first step in processing is the correct preparation of the developer and fixer solutions. For the best results, follow the manufacturer's directions exactly.

General precautions:

1) Make sure that the solutions are thoroughly mixed when prepared, and stirred before use each day.

2) Cover the developer tank with a lid to reduce contamination, evaporation and oxidation.

3) Replace solutions regularly. Discard solutions after three or four weeks, whether or not they have been used continuously. The use of processing solutions with diminished chemical activity can easily result in spoiled radiographs.

Temperature control

As the temperature of the processing solutions has a decided influence on their activity, careful control of this factor is essential. Laboratory tests indicate that the temperatures assuring satisfactory radiographic quality lie within a narrow range, the optimum value being 20°C (68°F). The table below gives the development times for KODAK Dental X-ray Films within the temperature range 18–24°C (64–75°F).

Developer	Dilution	Developing time at			
		18°C (64°F)	20°C (68°F)	22°C (72°F)	24°C (75°F)
Dental X-ray	1 + 4	5 min	4 min	3 min	2½ min
D-19	Undiluted	6 min	5 min	3¾ min	3 min
DX-80	1+4	5 min	4 min	3 min	2½ min
Rapid Dental X-ray	1+2		30 sec		

If the temperature of the developer is below that recommended, its action is retarded. If the temperature is too high, the rate of development increases. This may result in over-development, which can produce excessive fog, obscuring detail and decreasing contrast. In very warm solutions, the gelatin of the emulsion softens and becomes more liable to damage and, in extreme conditions, the emulsion may even melt and be washed off the support.

Preparation of film for processing

The first precaution in preparing film for processing, except when 'Defilux' Dental Film is being used, is to exclude all white light from the darkroom, in order to prevent fog. Only the light transmitted by the correct safelight filter is permissible. Open dental film packets carefully and place the films on a hanger, as shown in Figure 23. Slide extra-oral film into the hanger, as shown in Figure 24. Close the cassette immediately after removing the film, to avoid damage to the screens.

Processing procedure

Development

To begin processing, immerse the films in the developer and move them up and down several times in order to remove air bubbles that may have formed on the emulsion surfaces. To prevent films adhering to each other or to the sides of the tank, and to ensure that they are continually brought into contact with fresh developer, agitate the films at intervals throughout the developing period.

Rinse

After development, rinse the films for 10 seconds in a bath of clean water. If this stage is neglected, the fixing bath will become

Figure 23

Figure 24

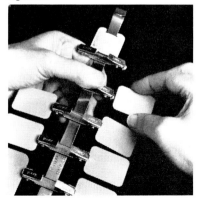
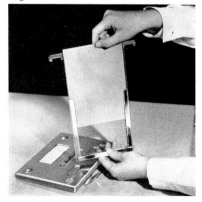

contaminated with developer carried over on the films and hangers, and will quickly become ineffective.

Fixing

Next, transfer the films to the fixing bath. During fixing, the films may be inspected occasionally by safelight to see when the silver halide has cleared from the emulsion. Keep the films in the fixing bath for at least twice the time taken for the film to clear, and not less than five minutes. The time required for fixing can be reduced if the films are agitated during this part of the process.

Washing

After fixing, wash the films in a bath of freely circulating running water for at least 10 minutes, to ensure the complete removal of fixing salts from the emulsion.

Drying

During the final stage, drying, the films must be handled with great care in order to avoid damage to the emulsion surface, which is particularly delicate when wet. Keep intra-oral films on their hangers during drying. Remove extra-oral films from their hangers after washing and hang them up to dry using film clips. A drip pan placed under the drying films is useful. Quick drying is usually desirable, and can be assisted by the use of an electric fan to circulate air round the films. For very rapid drying, the film may be dipped in 70 per cent surgical spirit after washing, but some deterioration of the surface may result.

Other information

Mounting intra-oral radiographs

Place the hanger with the complete set of radiographs flat on the bench, so that the various regions can be readily identified. Then place the radiographs in suitable mounts (these are obtainable from most dental supply houses).

In mounting a set of periapical radiographs, start with the upper central region and continue with the various regions in order of exposure, bearing in mind that all films of a series should be viewed from the same anatomical aspect. On KODAK Dental X-ray Films, the lingual aspect is identified by the depressed side of the embossed dot.

Filing radiographs

As an aid to future reference, radiographs should be filed with all the other case data. Identify radiographs by marking the name, date, and case number on the mounts before they are filed.

Typical faulty radiographs

Weak image

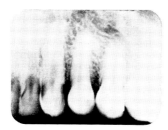

Possible causes:
Insufficient exposure to X-rays.
Insufficient development time.
Use of exhausted developer.
Developer temperature lower than recommended.
Incorrect dilution of the developer.

Dark image

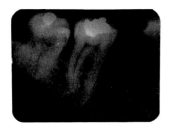

Possible causes:
Excessive exposure to X-rays.
Excessive development time.
Developer temperature higher than recommended.
Incorrect dilution of the developer.

Blurred image

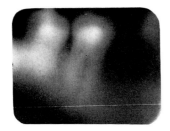

Possible causes:
Movement of the patient.
Movement of the film packet or cassette.
Movement of the X-ray tube.

Herringbone pattern

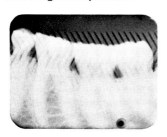

If a dental X-ray film is exposed with the back of the packet facing the X-ray tube the lead-foil backing will absorb a large amount of radiation during the exposure. This will result in a radiographic image that is of low density and low contrast. To distinguish between this and other possible causes of low density, the lead-foil backing used in KODAK Dental X-ray Film packets is embossed with a herringbone pattern, which is recorded on the film if it is exposed through the back.

Partial image

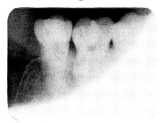

Possible causes:
Failure to direct the central ray at the centre of the film (1).

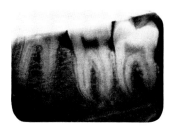

Developer level so low that only part of the film was immersed during processing (2).

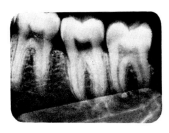

Two or more films were in contact during development (3).

Fog

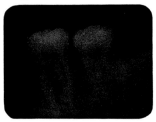

Fog always reduces radiographic contrast and makes interpretation more difficult.
Possible causes:
Storage of the film under adverse conditions.
Excessively prolonged storage of the film.
Exposure of the film to extraneous X-rays.
Exposure to white light.
Use of a faulty safelamp.
Use of the wrong safelight filter.
Excessively long development.
Development at very high temperatures.
Use of exhausted developer (see section on preparation of solutions, page 49).

Imperfectly mixed processing solutions (see same section).

Contamination of processing solutions by chemical deposits left in badly cleaned tanks.

Black line

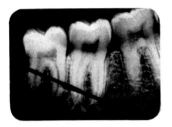

The straight black line is caused by excessive bending of the film.

Crimp mark

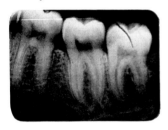

The crescent-shaped black line or crimp mark is caused by bending the corner of the film packet or by pressure from the nails on the emulsion when the film packet is being unwrapped.

Static marks

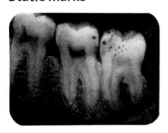

If an X-ray film is pulled too quickly from its wrapping when the atmosphere is dry, a charge of static electricity may be released. The film is blackened at the point of discharge and black marks radiate from this point.

Chemical splashes

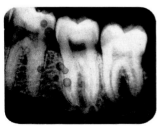

Developer or fixer, splashed on the film before processing, will produce blotches on the radiograph. Developer produces dark blotches, fixer clear ones.

Dark streaks

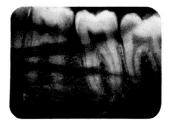

If dark streaks appear on a radiograph, it means that the clip has not been properly washed clean of fixer solution before being used again. The dried chemicals on the clip dissolve in the developer and run down the film.

Double exposure

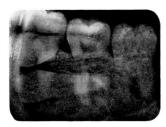

If film packets are placed on the bracket table or the operating cabinet after exposure, they may be picked up and used again. The result is that two exposures have to be re-made. Always place film packets in a lead-lined container immediately after exposure. This will also prevent fogging by extraneous X-rays.

Black specks

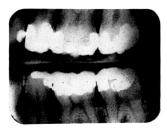

If an intra-oral film is not processed fairly promptly after exposure, moisture may penetrate the packet. Enclosure in a container with other damp packets will hasten this moisture penetration. In time the moisture may reach the inner black interleaving papers, which will then adhere to the film, leaving black particles on the surface when it is unwrapped.

Emulsion stripping

If a film is left in warm wash water for an excessively long period, for example, overnight, the emulsion may be softened to such an extent that it strips away from the film base.